Yorkshire

CW00719856

Contents

613 ᵘᵉ⁴

Health : Me

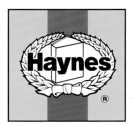

HAYNES PUBLISHING:
MORE THAN JUST MANUALS

Haynes Publishing Group is the world's market leader in the producing and selling of car and motorcycle repair manuals. Every vehicle manual is based on our experience of the vehicle being stripped down and rebuilt in our workshops. This approach, reflecting care and attention to detail, is an important part of all our publications. We publish many other DIY titles, as well as many books about motor sport, vehicles and transport in general.

Website: www.haynes.co.uk

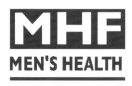

The Men's Health Forum's mini-manuals contain easy-to-read information covering a wide range of men's health subjects.
The Men's Health Forum's aim is to be an independent and respected promoter of male health, and to tackle the issues and problems affecting the health and well-being of boys and men in England and Wales.
Founded in 1994, The Men's Health Forum is a charity that works with a wide range of individuals and organisations to tackle male health issues. Well established and with an active membership, we work for the development of health services that meet men's needs and help men take more control of their own health and well-being. Our members, partners, staff and trustees bring plenty of experience in health care, media, business and activity.
Men's Health Forum, 32-36 Loman Street, London SE1 0EH
020 7922 7908
Website: www.menshealthforum.org.uk
Website: www.malehealth.co.uk
(for fast, free, independent health information from the Men's Health Forum)
Our registered office is as listed above.
A registered charity (number 1087375).
A company limited by guarantee (number 4142349 – England).

© Ian Banks 2009   *(009-12356)*
ISBN: 978 1 906121 75 4

Printed in the UK.

Haynes Publishing, Sparkford, Yeovil, Somerset BA22 7JJ, England

Haynes North America, Inc, 861 Lawrence Drive, Newbury Park, California 91320, USA

Haynes Publishing Nordiska AB, Box 1504, 751 45 Uppsala, Sweden

The author and the publisher have taken care to make sure that the advice given in this edition is right at the time of publication. We advise you to read and understand the instructions and information included with all medicines we recommend, and to carefully consider whether a treatment is worth taking. The author and the publisher have no legal responsibility for the results of treatments, misuse or over-use of the remedies in this book or their level of success in individual cases.
The author and the publisher do not intend this book to be used instead of advice from a medical practitioner, which you should always get for any symptom or illness.

Introduction

Yorkshire men are well known for many things, such as honesty, hard work, sport and especially straight-speaking. Unfortunately, men's health in Yorkshire is not as good as it could be. This mini-manual doesn't pretend to cover everything when it comes to perfect health, but it can make a difference along with common sense and better use of available health services. It's a no-nonsense guide to making informed choices about your health.

When all else fails, please read the instruction manual.

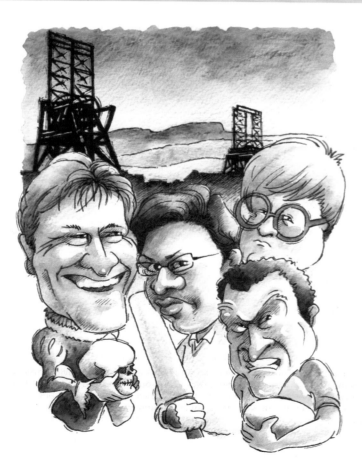

Getting active

Why bother?

Are you joking? It's not difficult to come up with excuses for being a couch potato, but there is now a huge amount of proof that exercise improves health in many different ways. If everyone walked for at least 30 minutes a day, five days a week, over one third of heart attacks could be prevented and thousands of lives could be saved each year.

What exercise can do for you

- As well as reducing your chances of having a heart attack, regular exercise can help prevent strokes, diabetes and some cancers. It can also improve blood pressure and cholesterol levels.
- It can help prevent osteoporosis (brittle bone disease), boost your immune system, give you more energy and even improve your sex life.
- It will make your muscles stronger and more flexible and make you less likely to suffer from depression.
- If you are overweight, your risk of heart disease is reduced if you exercise regularly, compared with people who are both overweight and unfit.

So you want to get fitter?

Your doctor is unlikely to tell you not to take more exercise. The important thing is to choose the right exercise for you and build up slowly.

Body basics

Choosing the right physical activity or exercise programme matters. If you aim for something too difficult you'll find yourself struggling to keep up, not to mention risk an injury.

- Go for gentle, easy exercise that you enjoy, then slowly build up.
- Don't try anything too difficult, and be realistic about what you can do.

Do what comes easiest

With this in mind, it is important that you choose exercise that you enjoy and that fits into your lifestyle. Just increasing the amount of activity in your everyday life can make a big difference. Try walking more by getting off the bus a stop earlier or parking the car further away from the shops or your workplace.

- Use the stairs rather than the lift or escalator.

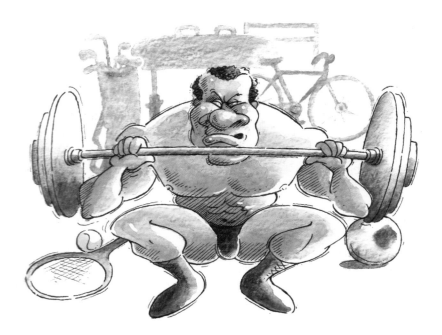

- Do more housework and all those DIY jobs you've been putting off.
- Go for as much variety as you can. If possible, go to the gym and play a sport.

You will be amazed how soon you feel better from simple exercise.

How much? How often? How hard?

You should exercise for around 30 minutes, five days a week. Although this may sound like a lot, you can break up the 30 minutes into two 15-minute or three 10-minute sessions. Any exercise that leaves you feeling slightly warmer and breathing more deeply counts.

Losing weight by exercising more is not easy and will take up to 60 minutes at least three times a week, on top of your 30 minutes of daily exercise. It's easier to lose weight by eating less than trying to burn it off through frantic exercise. And remember, exercise does more than just help you lose weight.

If you are very inactive don't panic, everyone has to start somewhere. Trying to do too much too soon will lead to you feeling exhausted and unlikely to keep going. It is better to aim for a slower, steady pace and keep going for longer than pushing yourself too hard when you start.

See **www.malehealth.co.uk/exercise.**

Weighty matters

So what's all the fuss about?

Eating a well-balanced diet can seriously improve your health by:
- keeping your weight down;
- lowering your blood cholesterol; and
- preventing high blood pressure.

All of these lower your risk of getting heart disease, which is the single biggest killer, and things like diabetes and cancer.

Boring? No chance

Eating well doesn't need to be boring. Eating a good variety of food makes sense and can be fun too. Basically you need:
- more fruit and vegetables;
- some starchy foods such as rice, bread, pasta and potatoes;
- less saturated fat, salt and sugar; and
- some protein-rich foods such as meat, fish, eggs and pulses.

Fruit and veg

Unless you have been hiding under a rock for the past few years you will know that eating plenty of fruit and vegetables is good for your health. Aim to eat at least five portions a day.

Fat facts

You do need some fat because it helps the body soak up some vitamins, it's a great energy boost and it supplies some of the things the body can't make itself. But too much fat means too much weight.
- Look for foods that are lower in fat.
- Try not to eat fatty foods too often.
- A plate of fried fish and chips won't kill you, but eating high fat foods all the time can seriously damage your health.
- Cut down on the fat you use in cooking. You should grill, casserole or stew meat instead of frying it.

Salt and increased blood pressure

Eating too much salt can raise your blood pressure, and people with high blood pressure are three times more likely to develop heart disease or have a stroke than people with normal blood pressure.

It's easy to build at least

5

different fruit and veg into your day.

One portion is:

1 medium glass of orange juice

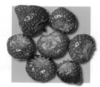
7 strawberries

A handful of sliced peppers, onions and carrots

1 medium apple

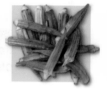
16 okra

1 medium banana

1 small mixed salad

3 heaped tablespoons of cooked kidney beans

3 whole dried apricots

3 heaped tablespoons of peas

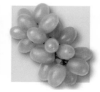
1 handful of grapes

1 tablespoon raisins

7 cherry tomatoes

3 heaped tablespoons of corn

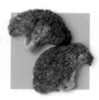
2 spears of broccoli

Tips to reduce salt
- Eat home-cooked meals rather than ready meals when possible.
- Use fresh turkey or chicken, fish and lean meat, rather than canned, smoked or processed meat.
- Go for food with low or reduced sodium levels or no added salt.
- Cook rice, pasta, and hot cereals without salt.
- Use herbs and spices instead of salt when cooking.

Heavyweight issues

Did you know that:
- obese people are 33% more likely to die from cancer than those who are a healthy weight;
- two out of every five people in the United Kingdom have high blood pressure;
- a person who is two stones overweight is twice as likely to have a heart attack as someone who is a healthy weight.
- every year, 30,000 deaths are directly linked to obesity, and every 17.5 minutes a person dies of an obesity-related illness. (Yorkshire and Humber has over 3,000 more deaths each year from obesity than the average figure for England); and
- by 2010, Yorkshire and Humber will top the charts for being the region with the highest percentage of obese men and women in England.

Good gut size

Men with a waist size of more than 94 centimetres (37 inches), or women with a waist bigger than 80 centimetres (32 inches), have increased health risks. A waist measurement of over 102 centimetres (40 inches) for men, or 88 centimetres (35 inches) for women, can lead to serious health risks.

African-Caribbean and Asian men have an increased risk of developing diabetes, high blood pressure and heart disease, and being overweight increases this risk. Being 40 years old is fine, having a 40-inch waist isn't.

How to measure your waist
- Find the top of your hip bone and the bottom of your ribs.
- Breathe out naturally.
- Place the tape measure between these points and wrap it around your waist.
- Make a note of the measurement.

See **www.malehealth.co.uk/diet.**

Coping with stress

Me, stressed? You cannot be serious!

Life without stress is impossible, and a small amount of stress can help, but a build-up of pressure can lead to a dangerous amount of stress. This can damage your health and even affect the people around you.

Most of us have experienced feelings such as being worried, being tense or feeling unable to cope. The good news is that there are things you can do to manage stress at home and especially at work, with support from those around you.

Stress signals

Although we all have to deal with stress, people vary in how much stress they can deal with before it has an effect on their life.

Watch out for common stress signals including:
- eating more or less than normal;
- mood swings;
- not being able to concentrate;
- feeling tense;
- feeling useless;
- feeling worried or nervous;
- not sleeping properly;
- being tired; and
- being forgetful.

Part of the problem is not recognising our own stress signals and expecting too much of ourselves.

Why bother?

Stress can trigger anxiety and depression and physical symptoms such as:
- back pain;
- indigestion;
- irritable bowel syndrome;
- psoriasis (scaly skin);
- migraine; and
- tension headaches.

There are several things you can do to help yourself and improve how you feel physically and mentally.

1 Time out

It can be hard to cope when you are feeling very stressed which is why it is important to take time out.

Quick fix

Getting yourself out of a stressful situation, even for a few moments, can give you the space you need to feel ready to tackle the problem.

Long term

Taking time out from your normal routine may help you deal with, and avoid, stress. If you have young children it is important to take a break. Try to organise a babysitter for an evening, or take it in turns with your partner to have time to yourselves. If you work:
- try to avoid doing long hours;
- take proper holidays; and
- take breaks away from your work area each day.

2   Work out

Exercise really helps you get rid of stress and prevents stress-related illness.

Quick fix

Go for a quick walk round the block to help you clear your head so you can deal with problems better.

Long term

Do at least 30 minutes of exercise a day (see pages 4 and 5). Try to build exercise into your daily routine (for example, you could cycle to work, walk to the shops, take the stairs instead of the lift, go for a walk and play games with your children).

3 Chill out

Getting enough sleep will relax your mind and help you cope with stress.

Quick fix

Simple relaxation techniques like breathing deeply can be an effective way of helping you deal with stress.

Long term

Plan relaxation time, even if it's just a long bath or listening to music.

Try to get a good night's sleep. Many people find relaxation techniques can be useful to help them cope. There are many types of relaxation classes available, such as meditation, yoga and Pilates. You should avoid sleeping tablets as they can be addictive and make things even worse.

4 Leave it out

Avoid smoking, junk food and alcohol! This won't help your stress levels. You should also avoid drinks that contain a lot of caffeine or sugar, as caffeine may make you feel more anxious and too much sugar can cause mood swings.

Quick fix

Drink plenty of water as this will help you concentrate and may stop you getting stress headaches.

Long term

Improving your diet and drinking plenty of water will help your body to deal with stress. It's important to make time for proper meals to keep your energy levels high. Talk during meals as this is a time to relax as well as eat.

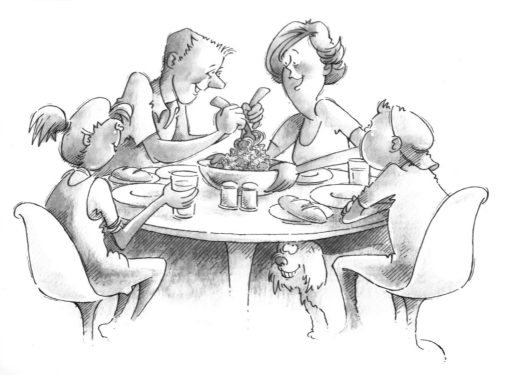

5 *Talk it out*

Just talking about things that are making you stressed may help you see things differently. It can help you find a way of tackling practical problems that may be causing stress.

Talk to your friends or family

Dealing with stress alone is never a good idea. Talking to even one other person can help you deal with stress, and family or friends may be able help you.

Talk with colleagues

It may be hard to believe but work is generally good for our well-being. At times, though, it can be stressful. Men tend not to want to talk about problems at work, but it might be helpful to chat with your mates.

These days, most employers want to hear of problems before they lose a valuable employee. Trade unions also have staff specially trained to deal with stress at work. Find out if your company has a counselling or occupational health service.

Talk with a health professional

You can speak to a doctor or practice nurse for advice and support, or contact NHS Direct (see **Contacts** at the back). You can also ask at a chemist for advice.

See **www.malehealth.co.uk/stress.**

Sensible drinking

Keeping to the limits

Lower risk drinking means no more than three to four units a day for men and two to three units a day for women. If you keep to these amounts, in most circumstances, you should prevent damaging your health. If you already do this you don't need to take any action, just carry on being aware of what you drink and remember that it's easy to drink more than this without really noticing.

If you regularly drink more than you should (over 35 units a week for men or 21 units for women) you might already have experienced problems like feeling tired or depressed, putting on weight, memory loss when drinking, sleeping badly and having sexual problems. You could also suffer from high blood pressure. Some people are argumentative if they drink a lot, and this can have a negative effect on their relationships with family and friends.

Easy does it

Just how heavy is your drinking?			
Large glass of wine (175 millilitres)	15%	3 units	120 to 170 calories
Small glass of wine (125 millilitres)	12%	1½ units	85 to 120 calories
Bottle of wine (750 millilitres)	12%	9 units	255 to 360 calories
Pint of beer	5%	3 units	180 calories
Pint of beer	3.5%	2 units	160 to 170 calories
Single measure of spirits (25 millilitres)	40%	1 unit	60 to 75 calories

The amount of alcohol in your blood after a certain number of drinks depends on the following.
- Body weight – the percentage of alcohol in your bloodstream will depend on your size and weight.
- Body fat – alcohol is absorbed more slowly if you have extra body fat, but can also make you put more weight on.
- What is in your stomach – fatty foods can make your body absorb alcohol more slowly.

Alcohol also affects you differently depending on the following.
- The time of day – early drinking has a bigger effect.
- How rested you are – being stressed can make things worse.
- Medicines – always read the label. If you're not sure, don't drink alcohol when you are taking medicines without first asking your doctor or pharmacist.

Hangovers

A bad hangover can make you feel extremely ill. If you do find yourself with a hangover, drink plenty of water, take some paracetamol as shown on the bottle and, if possible, have a nap later in the day to make up for the poor quality of your sleep. You won't be able to do this if you are at work and this is why drinking too much alcohol affects your ability to work and increases the risk of accidents.

Hangovers are not usually dangerous unless you have too many. Don't have an alcoholic drink to ease a hangover as this can lead to alcohol abuse.

Should I try to cut down on my drinking?

Are you surprised or shocked to find yourself in the increasing-risk or higher-risk category? If you are in one of these categories, you need to lower your alcohol intake and put a stop to the harm you're doing to your health. For more information go to **www.units.nhs.uk** or call 0800 917 8282.

Most people just need to cut down on their drinking, but there are some people who need to stop completely.

If you're in the lower-risk category, you probably don't need to take any action, although you may still need to cut down. You should always keep an eye on your drinking, and keep this booklet in case you need it in the future.

Drinking tips

- Walk to the pub to burn off some extra calories on the way.
- Drink plenty of water, both during the day and when drinking alcohol.
- Try to drink after a meal instead of before – you won't spoil your appetite and you won't feel like drinking so much after your meal.
- Try reducing the strength of what you drink. For example, if you drink 5% beer, try 3.5% beer instead.
- Try to have at least one alcohol-free day a week.
- Do things with friends or family that don't involve drinking. For example, meet up for a sports session, or go to the cinema instead.

See **www.malehealth.co.uk/drinking.**

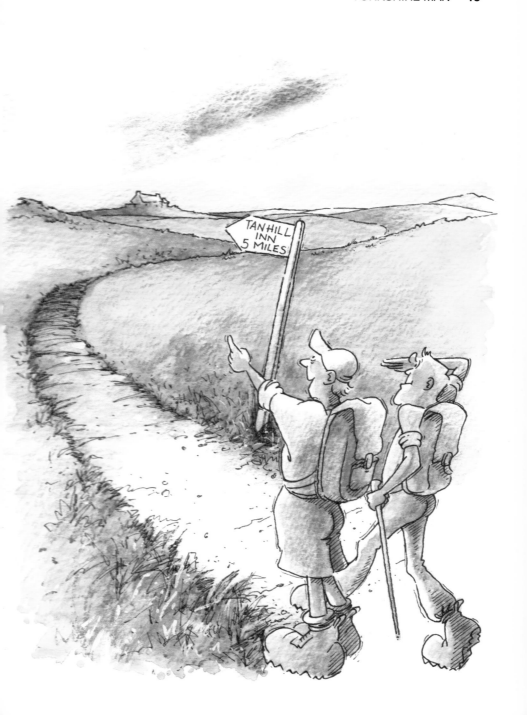

No smoke without fire

As many as seven out of 10 smokers want to quit. Stopping smoking could be the best thing you'll ever do in your life. It can be a life-changing experience. Stop smoking and look forward to years of better health.

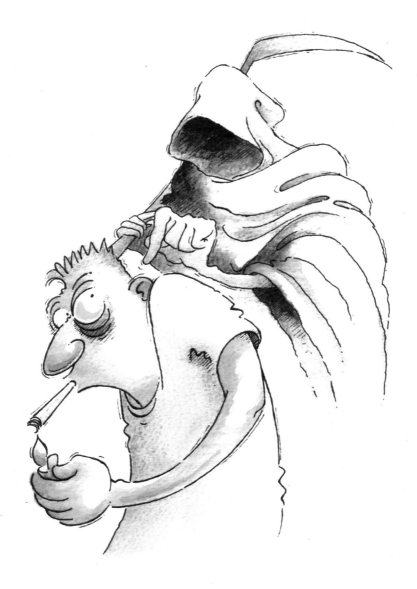

Stopping smoking is the one single thing you can do to massively increase your chances of living longer. Once you've stopped smoking, your body will begin to heal within 20 minutes, repairing the damage done by all those years of smoking.

- After 20 minutes your blood pressure and pulse will return to normal. Your circulation will improve – especially in your hands and feet.
- After eight hours your blood oxygen levels will return to normal and your risk of having a heart attack will fall.
- After 24 hours carbon monoxide will leave your body. Your lungs will also start to clear out mucus and smoke-related rubbish.
- After 48 hours your body will be nicotine-free, and your sense of taste and smell will improve.
- After 72 hours you will breathe easier and you will have more energy.
- After two to 12 weeks your circulation will improve, and it will be easier for you to walk and do exercise.
- After three to nine months your breathing problems will improve. You can say goodbye to coughing, shortness of breath and wheezing.
- After five years of not smoking your risk of having a heart attack will have halved.

Facts about smoking

- Smoking harms nearly every organ in the body, causing many diseases and reducing your quality of life and how long you live.
- Smoking causes, bronchitis, emphysema, heart disease, lung cancer and cancer in other organs including the lip, mouth, throat, bladder, kidney, stomach and liver.
- Breathing in other people's cigarette smoke can also cause these diseases. It is never safe to breathe in other people's smoke.
  To protect yourself and your family from this you should ban smoking in your home and your car and avoid smoking in public places.
- One in two long-term smokers will die early as a result of smoking – half of these in middle age.
- Smoking is also linked to erection problems.

Lighting-up times

Do you want to stop smoking but you're not sure how to do it? Preparing to stop smoking is about being practical and having a plan. People stop smoking every day, and you can too.

How do I stop?
- Contact your local NHS Stop Smoking Service – a free service where trained experts are waiting to help you. You can talk to an adviser or share your experiences as part of a group.
- Sign up to the Together Program by contacting the NHS Smoking Helpline.
- Use nicotine-replacement products such as patches, gum and inhalators to cope with your withdrawal symptoms and cravings.
- People who use medication and get professional help to stop smoking can double their chances of success.

Planning to quit
- Set a day to stop smoking.
- Work out what encourages or tempts you to smoke and plan ahead to avoid these situations.
- Tell all your friends and relatives so they can help you.
- Take it one day at a time and reward yourself every day.
- Find a friend who wants to stop smoking so you can support each other.
- Avoid situations where you might be tempted to smoke.
- Clear the house and your pockets of any cigarette packets, papers or matches.
- Keep track of your progress on a chart or calendar.
- Keep the money you saved in a separate container.
- Ask your friends not to smoke around you.
- Keep telling yourself you can do it.
- Don't just rely on willpower alone.

See **www.malehealth.co.uk/smoking.**

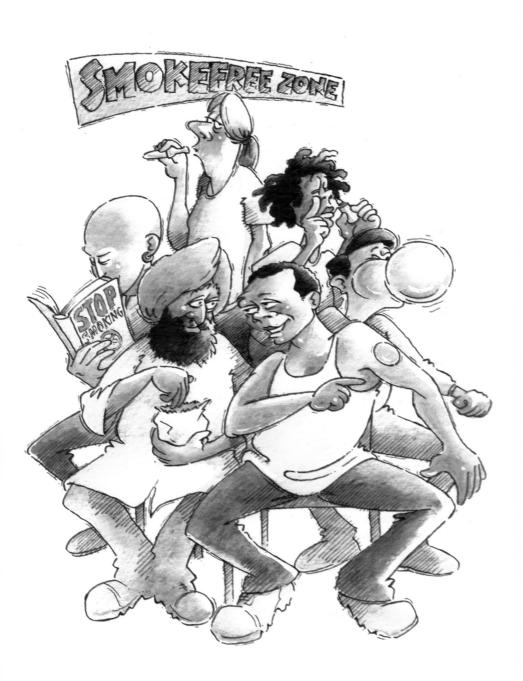

Mouth matters

Men visit their dentist less often than women, but most things that go wrong in your mouth can be prevented.

Bad teeth (dental decay)

Sugary or starchy foods or drinks feed bacteria which naturally live in the mouth. This then produces acids which can rot your teeth. An unhealthy mix of food, bacteria and saliva called 'plaque' builds up around teeth, attacking the tough enamel on the outside. If left, this will destroy the teeth.

Prevention

Brushing with a fluoride toothpaste every night and morning, and avoiding sugary drinks or food, will help prevent bad teeth. Bad teeth only start to hurt once they are badly damaged, so see your dentist at least every year for a check-up. Go to the dentist straightaway if you have:

- toothache or sensitivity to hot, cold or sweet things;
- discoloured spots on your teeth;
- bad breath; or
- an unpleasant taste in your mouth.

Plaque

To really get rid of plaque you need to regularly replace your toothbrush.

- Buy a new brush at least every couple of months.
- Circular brushing is best for the side teeth. Use downwards brush strokes away from the gums at the front.
- Back teeth (molars) need brushing backwards and forwards.

Tooth tips

Go for teeth-friendly foods such as:

- cheese (in moderation);
- vegetables;
- sugar-free gum; and
- unsweetened tea, coffee or soft drinks.

Bad breath (halitosis)

Bad breath is very common but it can be difficult to realise that you have it. It takes a very good friend to tell you that you have bad breath.

Some foods cause smelly breath (onions are a good example), but the smell should go away very soon. The most common causes of bad breath are bad teeth, gum infections or chest infections.

Treatment

It depends on the cause, but in most cases regular brushing will get rid of bad breath.

> *Breath hints*
> - Brush at least twice a day.
> - Eat a healthy, balanced diet.
> - Don't drink too much alcohol.
> - Stop smoking.
> - Use a mouthwash, but only one recommended by your dentist or pharmacist.
> - Drink plenty of water.
> - Chew sugar-free gum after eating, and if your mouth feels dry.
> - Avoid sugary food and snacks.
> - See your dentist at least once a year.

Do you have trouble finding an NHS dentist? See **www.nhs.uk.**

Mouth ulcers

These can really be a pain, especially when eating or drinking. Sometimes there seems to be no cause, but you should watch out for:
- brushing your teeth too hard;
- badly-fitting dentures;
- anxiety and stress;
- some foods such as chocolate, coffee, peanuts, almonds, strawberries, cheese, tomatoes and wheat flour; and
- not eating enough vitamin B12. Try eating yeast extract – if it works you know what the problem is.

Treatment

You can get rid of most ulcers with some corticosteroid cream or a mouthwash from your pharmacist. You should see your doctor if there is no improvement after a few days.

Mouth cancer

Men are much more likely than women to develop mouth cancer, usually on the tongue, lips or gums. Watch out for:
- a lump or sore on the lip or in the mouth which doesn't go away after a few weeks; and
- lumps or pains in the neck.

Most mouth cancer is caused by smoking (and chewing tobacco) and can be made worse with too much alcohol. The good news is that mouth cancer can be cured, but only if caught early, so regular checks with your dentist are a good idea.

Healthy bones

Bone is an actively growing organ that is constantly adapting to stresses and strains on the body. Long periods of weightlessness in space lead to a gradual reduction in bone strength. This is also seen at a lower level in people who cannot get out of bed or don't do much exercise. Regular exercise is very important in keeping the spine strong and flexible.

But exercise alone is not enough to keep the balance right – what you eat is just as important. You need to eat the right food, but not too much of it, as being overweight is one of the major causes of back problems because it reduces activity and flexibility and also puts added strain on the muscles, ligaments and bones.

It is a myth that only children need lots of calcium to build their bones.
Adults' bones are constantly changing and being renewed and need plenty of calcium. The body can only store this important mineral in the bone itself, so you need fresh calcium every day. The best way to get calcium is from dairy products such as milk, cheese, yogurt, bread and the bones you can eat from fish such as sardines. Green leafy vegetables provide vitamins and calcium and help to protect you from heart disease and cancer.

Sunshine vitamins

It's not enough just to eat plenty of calcium as the body needs vitamin D to help take it in from the stomach. Sunlight converts an inactive form of vitamin D into the type which does this. You need a healthy balance between too much sun (which can cause skin cancer) and too little (which can cause bones to become thinner).

Bone building

Bones are denser when you are between 25 and 30 years old. Bones need you to do weight-bearing exercise to prevent them from thinning and not being flexible. Weight-bearing exercises include gardening, walking fast, sport, dancing and housework. Giving up smoking also helps keep bones strong and flexible.

Back care

A painful back is one of life's miseries and because other people cannot 'see' the pain it gets little sympathy. 'Bad backs' are also one of the greatest causes of sickness-related absence from work. More than 90% of people will suffer from back problems at some time in their life and for many it will be a constant cause of discomfort or pain.

The spine

There are 33 bones in the spine. Small joints give the spine flexibility without damaging the spinal cord which runs through it. Over-stretching or injury to the spine can lead to severe pain and even loss of movement in the limbs.

Nervous road map

All messages to and from the brain pass through the spine. Injury or too much strain will lead to reduced flexibility and cause back pain. We take the spine for granted until it reacts to being treated badly. Serious back pain can be caused by bad posture, not lifting things properly or accidental injury, and these can all make problems you may already have even worse.

Muscle problems

Your back is supported by hundreds of different muscles, including those that also support the arms, legs and head. These range from the really strong muscles seen on your back to those inside the body, all of which can be strained or overworked, leaving the spine at risk of damage. Most back pain comes from injured muscle or muscle tendons rather than the spine itself. When hurt, muscle can spasm and be unable to relax properly, and this leads to more pain and possibly more damage so it is important to rest straightaway. You should exercise gently as the injury settles rather than stay too long in bed, as being upright is always better than lying down.

Back to basics – self-care

Advice on the best way to treat a bad back changes all the time. Exercise, not bed rest, is now considered best. Serious back pain may need rest or to be checked by a doctor.

Try to reduce the pressure on the spine when lying down. It can help to lie sideways with your legs slightly bent and with a cushion between them. Tension is part of the problem and a gentle back massage can be really effective. Don't stay in the same position too long – roll over or even stand up and walk for a few steps. A mix of non-steroidal anti-inflammatory medicines (for example, ibuprofen) and paracetamol can really help (always follow the instructions on the packet).

Swapping between warm towels and cool compresses can help relax muscles and reduce inflammation. As the pain reduces, try to move around as normal but avoid lifting anything or straining your back.

You should call NHS Direct (0845 46 47) if you have:

- serious pain in either or both your legs;
- a loss of feeling or power in your legs; or
- trouble urinating.

Back to the future

Bad backs are no joke and they really can hurt more when you laugh.
To avoid a bad back you need to lift things in the right way, have better
posture and look after your bones, muscles, tendons and ligaments. When
things go wrong you need to ignore medical myths and follow current
advice. A gentle return to full activity is better than weeks of lying in bed
with a door under the mattress.

See **www.malehealth.co.uk/back.**

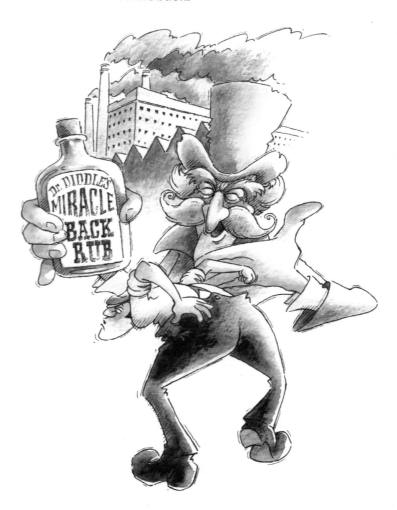

Sexual health

Sexually transmitted infections (STIs)

The best way to prevent sexually transmitted infections is to practise safer sex. Use a condom whenever you have sex, because STIs can be a serious problem. They can affect you at any age, whether you're straight or gay, in a long-term relationship or with a casual partner. Symptoms don't always show up immediately, so you could have been infected recently or a long time ago. If you have had unsafe sex or are at all worried, you can have a confidential check-up, and treatment if needed, at a genitourinary medicine (GUM) or STI clinic.

Although extra lubrication is sometimes needed, do not use oil-based lubricants such as petroleum jelly or baby oil with condoms, as they will damage the condom (as can lipstick!). There are water-based lubricants available, but if you are not sure, ask your chemist as they will not be embarrassed to give you advice.

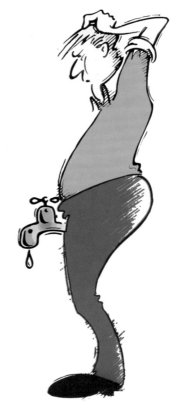

Prostate problems

Only men have a prostate gland. It's round and about the size of a golf ball. It is in the pelvis, against the base of the bladder. The prostate surrounds the urethra – the tube that runs from your bladder inside your penis to the outside (you urinate through it). Imagine the prostate as a fat rubber washer around a bit of tubing. It grows to adult size during puberty. In most men it also begins to grow again in early middle age, which can cause problems. (These problems are common.)

There are two possible causes of an enlarged prostate: benign prostate hyperplasia (BPH) – a benign (non-cancerous) enlargement of the prostate gland common in men over 50 – and prostate cancer. The symptoms are very similar and are usually related to problems urinating, such as the following.

- A constant need to urinate, especially at night.
- Rushing to the toilet.
- Difficulty starting to urinate.
- Difficulty urinating.
- Taking a long time urinating.
- Having a weak flow of urine.
- Feeling that your bladder has not emptied properly.
- Dribbling after you've finished urinating.
- Pain or discomfort when urinating.

Other symptoms can include the following.

- Lower back pain.
- Pain in your pelvis, hips or thighs.
- Erection problems.
- Blood in the urine – this is rare.
- Pain when you ejaculate.
- Pain in your penis or testicles.

It is important that you know that any of these symptoms can also be caused by problems which are nothing to do with prostate cancer. If you are concerned about any symptoms that you have, visit your doctor.

Enlarged prostate (BPH)

BPH rarely causes symptoms before the age of 40, but more than half of men in their sixties and as many as 90% in their seventies and eighties have some symptoms of BPH.

As the prostate enlarges, tissue layers surrounding it prevents it from growing evenly, and pressure then squashes the urethra like a clamp on a garden hose. As a result, the bladder wall becomes thicker and irritated, shrinking even when it contains small amounts of urine, causing you to urinate more often. The bladder will eventually weaken and lose the ability to empty itself, trapping urine inside. The urethra becoming narrower and the bladder not emptying completely cause many of the problems linked with BPH. Some men with very enlarged prostates might not suffer while others with less-enlarged prostates can have more problems.

The problem can be treated with drugs or by surgically removing the enlarged part of the prostate. There is a small risk that either treatment may cause impotence (being unable to get and keep an erection) but you can speak to your doctor about this.

Prostate cancer

Older men of African or Caribbean origin are at high risk of getting prostate cancer. Men who have had a close male blood relative, especially a brother, with prostate cancer also seem to have an increased risk of getting it.

The Western diet of highly refined food with a high animal fat content also seems to increase the risk of developing prostate cancer. There is no firm evidence of how to reduce the risk of prostate cancer. We do know that having a healthy diet with more fruit and vegetables, less red meat and more fish is good for reducing the risks of other cancers, heart disease and possibly prostate cancer.

It is important to be clear – not all men get symptoms that show they have prostate cancer. In the men that do, not all men have exactly the same symptoms. You do not have to have all the symptoms listed to have prostate cancer.

Prostate cancer is treated in several different ways, and it can depend on how aggressive the cancer is, whether it has spread elsewhere in your body and how old you are. Your general state of health may also make a difference.

You can speak to your doctor about your options.

You may be able to reduce your risk with the occasional Bloody Mary, preferably with more tomato juice than vodka. Tomatoes are said to protect you.

Testicular cancer

Testicular problems are quite rare, and testicular cancer is the most serious. It represents only 1% of all cancers in men, but it is the single biggest cause of cancer-related death in men aged between 18 and 35.

Symptoms of testicular cancer
- A lump on one testicle.
- Pain and tenderness in either testicle.
- Discharge (pus or smelly goo) from the penis.
- Blood in the sperm when you ejaculate.
- A build-up of fluid inside the testicular sac (scrotum).
- A heavy dragging feeling in the groin or scrotum.
- An increase in the size of a testicle.
- An enlargement of the breasts, with or without tenderness.

Preventing testicular cancer
For once, men are positively encouraged to check themselves, but this time to do more than just 'check they're still there'. Self-examination is the

name of the game. Check your testicles every month in the following ways.

- Do it lying in a warm bath or while having a long shower, as this makes the skin of the scrotum softer.
- Hold the scrotum in the palm of your hand and feel the difference between the testicles. You will very probably feel that one is larger and lying lower, which is completely normal.
- Examine each one in turn, and then compare them with each other. Use both hands and gently roll each testicle between your thumb and forefinger. Check for any lumps or swellings as they should both be smooth. Remember that the duct carrying sperm to the penis, the epididymis, normally feels bumpy. It lies along the top and back of the testis.

Checking your testicles too often can actually make it more difficult to notice any difference and may cause unnecessary worry.

Erectile Dysfunction (an inability to get or keep an erection)

Problems with erections are common. At least one in 10 British men have had some sort of erection problems at some stage in their lives and around one man in 20 has permanent erection problems. This is not helped by most men not wanting to talk about these problems, despite the fact that virtually all erection problems can be sorted out with simple treatments.

It is very important to find out what is causing the problem as diabetes and high blood pressure are commonly linked conditions.

At one time, what a man was thinking about was considered the major factor for erection problems. We now know that around one-third of all cases will be due to psychological issues and can often respond well to non-clinical treatments such as sex counselling. Normally, if you have erections at any time other than during attempted intercourse you have a psychological rather than physical problem. Getting an erection during television programmes, sexy videos or self-masturbation is a good sign, although it is not a 100% test.

See **www.malehealth.co.uk/sexualhealth**

Getting the best from the NHS

Don't get caught in the web

Buying drugs from illegal internet sites is potentially very dangerous. Almost all such drugs are at best fake and useless, at worst harmful. You may also have your credit card details stolen as well. More important is the danger of not getting a medical diagnosis. Erection problems won't kill you but linked diabetes or high blood pressure most certainly can. You should speak your doctor or chemist about this first.

More than ever before, the NHS has a range of services that offer convenient options that allow you to get the right treatment at the right time, and at the right place. These services can make life a lot easier so visit **www.nhsdirect.nhs.uk** or phone 0845 46 47.

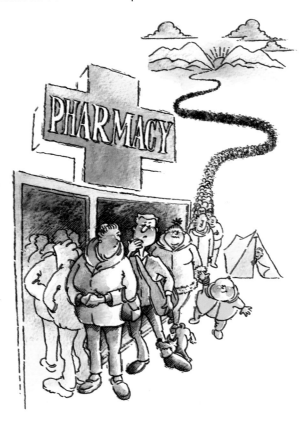

Pharmacists: more than just blue bottles

Pharmacists are highly qualified professionals providing advice on the use and selection of prescription and over-the-counter (OTC) medicines. They can give advice on how to manage small problems and common conditions. This includes lifestyle advice about eating habits, exercise and stopping smoking but they will also tell you where you can get advice from.

NHS Walk-in Centres: a step in the right direction

Highly qualified NHS nurses offer a range of convenient and free services, with no need to make an appointment. They also offer good advice, look after minor illnesses and injuries, provide prescriptions and even provide emergency contraception. Look out for the centres in railway stations, shopping centres or on the high street. They normally open from 7am until 10pm, Monday to Friday, and
9am to 10pm, Saturday and Sunday.

NHS Direct: direct and to the point

NHS Direct provides 24-hour confidential health advice and information. Phone 0845 46 47 or visit NHS Direct Online at **www.nhsdirect.nhs.uk**. Why not try NHS Direct Interactive on digital satellite TV?

Doctors' surgeries

Doctors are often available from around 8.30am to 6pm (or later). Calling at other times will put you in touch with an out-of-hours system. It's always best to see your own doctor if possible, so unless your problem is urgent and cannot wait, you should make an appointment to be seen by your normal doctor. Practices now often offer a huge range of services such as minor surgery, skincare, chiropody and even diabetic clinics.

Getting the best from your doctor

If you don't turn up for an appointment you can cause huge frustration, especially because you haven't had any medical attention.

You should:
- Write down your symptoms before you see your doctor. It's extremely easy to forget the most important things during the examination. Doctors will spot important clues about a problem, by asking questions

like when did the problem start and how did it feel? Did anyone else suffer as well? Has this ever happened before? What have you done about it so far? Are you taking any medicine for it?

- Ask questions, and don't be afraid to ask your doctor to give more information or make something clear that you don't understand. Asking them to write it down for you is a good idea.
- Get to the point – if you have a lump or bump say so. Time is limited so there is a real danger of you coming out with a prescription for a sore nose when you might need a serious problem sorted.
- Have your prescription explained, and ask whether you can buy any medicines from your chemist. Make sure you know what each medicine is for. Some medicines clash badly with alcohol.

Dentists

You will have to pay for dental check-ups and treatment unless you are at school, are pregnant or receive certain benefits. To find an NHS dentist in your area, go to **www.nhs.uk.**

Accident and emergency

Accident and emergency departments treat serious accidents or life-threatening illnesses such as heart attacks or medical conditions which suddenly become worse. They are open 24 hours a day all year, and are often used by people who should really see their own doctor or a pharmacist. You should be prepared to wait if there are people more seriously ill than you.